By

Annika Reinert

© 2018 Annika Reinert

ISBN: 9781717863997

BETTER & HEALTHY
LIFE
BY ANNIKA REINERT

CHAPTER ONE 1

   FITNESS FOR MEN OVER 50 1
   WEIGHT LOSS FOR MEN OVER 50 CANNOT BE ACCOMPLISHED THROUGH INCREASED ACTIVITY ALONE 5
   WEIGHT LOSS ROUTINE STEPS FOR MEN OVER 50 YEARS 12
   MY DIETARY SUPPLEMENTS FOR MEN OVER 50 WANTING BETTER HEALTH 15

CHAPTER TWO 22

   NUTRITION AND ADEQUATE PROTEIN INTAKE FOR WEIGHT LOSS FOR MEN OVER 50 22
   MUSCLE BUILDING FOR MEN - ADVICE AND TIPS 25

CHAPTER THREE 28

   WORKOUT FOR MEN OVER 50 28
   Fitness For Men Over 50 - Workout Routines For Obese Men Aged 50 Plus to Burn Fat and Lose Weight 31

CHAPTER FOUR 37

   CLEAN EATING WORKOUT NUTRITION PLAN FOR MEN OVER 50 37

CHAPTER FIVE 42

   MUSCLE BUILDING, FITNESS AND DIET MYTHS 42

CHAPTER SIX 50

   WEIGHTLIFTING AND EGO IN YOUR 50'S AND BEYOND 50

CHAPTER SEVEN 57

   WORKOUT PLAN FOR MEN OVER 50 57

CHAPTER EIGHT 66

   FASTEST WAY TO GAIN MUSCLE 66

CHAPTER NINE 74

   TIPS ON DIET AND EXERCISE FOR MEN 74
   VITAMINS AND MINERALS FOR THE OVER 50'S 83

CHAPTER TEN 90

   WHAT ARE THE NECESSARY THING TO CONSIDER FOR MEN OVER 50 90

CHAPTER ONE

FITNESS FOR MEN OVER 50

If you are wondering if there are foods that complement your men's fitness program, the answer is Yes.

But before I even discuss the foods, you should be prepared about the different advices that you receive about eating from various sources. There are nutritionists who advice eating in smaller meals of about 6 to 8 times daily. Some nutritionists advise eating three regular meals every day. There is so many advice that most people end up getting confused.

Well, one thing is for sure, 'one size fits all' is not applicable to fitness for men over 50. Body composition varies from one man to another so the times that you have to eat will depend on your requirements and fitness goals.

It would be best to stick to the basic if you are not sure what to do. Eat three full meals i.e. breakfast, lunch and dinner. You may also have a light snack in between if you want.

Going back to the question, what are the specific foods that may complement your workout and help you achieve optimal results?

1: Protein

Protein is an essential nutrient for your fitness diet as it increases the metabolic rate of the body. A higher metabolic rate basically means getting fit faster and easier. Apart from that, protein also helps in building leaner and stronger muscles. Some sources of protein include lean meat like chicken, beef, turkey, pork, and lamb. Tuna, eggs and walnut are also rich in protein.

Knowing to eat, the right types of meat is equally crucial to knowing how to cook them. The best way to cook them is grilling instead of frying. If for some reason you still have to fry the meat, you will need oil and seasoning. It would be better to add olive oil as it contains healthy fat. The same goes with seasoning wherein it should contain less sugar otherwise your fitness goals will be defeated. Avoid marinating your meat as much as possible, especially those that contain brown sugar and corn syrup.

2: Fresh vegetables

Fitness gurus will definitely tell you the importance of eating fresh vegetables. Vegetables contain vitamins that are needed for the body to function properly. Vegetables also contain fiber which helps in improving digestion.

There are many vegetables to choose from and include in your fitness for men program. The more colors you incorporate, the better. Beans, squash, tomatoes and bell peppers are some of the most nutritious vegetables.

Vegetables can be eaten raw but if you want to cook them, prefer grilling over boiling or steaming as the last two cooking processes take away the nutrient contents of the vegetable.

3: Fresh fruits

Vegetables and fresh fruits go hand in hand. There is an emphasis on 'fresh' because canned fruits contain high levels of sugar, which is harmful to the body.

Fresh fruit choices are endless from apples, peach, pineapple, pear, banana to different kinds of berries like strawberry and blueberry.

These were the three food groups that is highly recommended in our fitness program. On the other hand, there are food groups that you must avoid:

4: Dairy products

While dairy products are beneficial, some contain fats and sugar. You have to avoid eating these unless you are under a highly intense fitness program, and are performing fitness exercises that can compensate for the consumption of the extra fat.

Dairy products that you should limit are milk, yogurt and cheese.

5: Particular carbohydrate-rich foods

Some foods rich in carbohydrates are usually loaded with sugar and empty calories. These are mainly starches which are converted into fat when stored in the body. The fat converting process could be more profound if you are living a sedentary lifestyle.

Some of these carbohydrate-rich foods are pasta, rice, bread, cereal and potatoes. Fried carbohydrates like French fries and hash browns are even more harmful the body and must be completely avoided.

WEIGHT LOSS FOR MEN OVER 50 CANNOT BE ACCOMPLISHED THROUGH INCREASED ACTIVITY ALONE

Men over 50 are typical at the busiest time of their lives. Work and family responsibilities, often spreading over two generations by this time, and adding even modest amounts of time to daily schedule is not realistic.

The answer of course is that the problem can not be solved only by increasing activity. Healthy activity should be part of the lives of men over 50, and this argument assumes that is taking place. The study, however, spoke of substantial increases in activity levels and still not being able to reverse thickening waist lines.

Weight gain with age happens because as we age we lose lean muscle mass. With the loss of lean muscle mass, all other factors being equal, our RMR, or resting metabolic rate, decreases too. This is part of the physiological changes that take place as we age that make weight loss for men over 50 an increasing challenge.

The solution is in nutrition. It is possible for men over 50 to build lean muscle mass and the key is feeding the body what it needs. The habits built up over the previous fifty or more years probably won't promote the creation and maintenance of lean muscle mass even in men who have been attentive to their diet and nutrition.

Since metabolism in men over 50 slows, basic caloric intake should be reduced as well. There is not a "one size fits all" solution to this calculation because it depends on current weight and activity level. Maintaining lean muscle mass through nutrition and ongoing healthy activity is the way men over 50 can support a trim and healthy physique.

Easy to Follow Workouts Routine For 50 Plus Men to Lose Weight

Weight loss for men over 50 is possible provided they take up easy and natural methods. After reaching this age it becomes all the more necessary for an individual to opt for simple methods which would keep him fit and at the same time help him to lose weight quite easily. In such, a case one can opt for easy workout routines which can help 50 plus men to lose weight at a very steady pace.

Before indulging in any workout routine, you must check out the following factors like whether you are a smoker or whether you are suffering from high blood pressure or high cholesterol level. You are compelled to check out these factors in order to pick up those workouts only which would not affect your body.

Here are some easy workouts for men to lose weight

Start your workout with a 5 min warm-up i.e., either by cycling or running on a treadmill. Then start with the boxing rounds provided you don't forget to take 30 seconds rest in between.

During the second step you can opt for pushups. Do as many times as you want within the allotted time i.e., 2 minutes.

* After that you can switch over to the jump rope. In this case your shoulders might experience some pain but it would let out the lactic acid. Here your lungs will also hurt but it would provide you a good feeling.

Then after 30 seconds rest you can move onto intensive workout with the support of jump rope.

In this step you must get onto our knees and carry out two minutes of exercise in ab wheel. This exercise would make your shoulders and back very strong. After that take rest for 30 seconds.

Now grab 10 or 15 lb dumbbells and make your shoulders work by pressing the dumbbell. Do this workout for at least 2 minutes.

Lastly, grab the jump rope once again and start doing intensive rope work for two minutes

5 Benefits Of Walking On A Treadmill For Men Over 50

Trying to keep up with an exercise routine is difficult in your younger years and doesn't get any easier as we get older. As you age, you begin to feel strange things happening to your body. All of a sudden you have sore and aching joints, various medical problems develop and you notice a general lack of energy.

Your doctor will tell you that exercise is what you need to start feeling more energetic and stronger, to help keep your blood pressure down and to improve your overall attitude.

Even if you haven't been working out or exercising for a few years and regardless of the condition you are in now. You can start a walking exercise program, and I suggest that you start out on a treadmill. Treadmills provides an easy and convenient way to exercise regardless of weather conditions and in the comfort and safety of your own home.

Since I have started walking on a treadmill as my exercise routine, I have discovered some great benefits.

Here are 5 benefits of using a treadmill that I would like to share with you.

Benefit 1

Walking on a treadmill will not harm or aggravate sore joints.

Even if you have arthritis, inflamed joints, or problems with your feet. For those of you that like to walk on your streets, you know that the pounding you take on the concrete will make your joints hurt, and discourage you from another workout.

Treadmills have soft, padded walking areas so you can workout longer and improve your fitness quicker.

Benefit 2

You Can Improve Your Cardiovascular Health

Walking is considered to be one of the best cardiovascular exercises for men over the age of 50. It doesn't matter what your body type is, your fitness level or your exercise history. Walking is a basic form of aerobic training and has many benefits for the heart, lungs, and circulatory system. Treadmill walking will also increase muscle tone and burn fat calories.

Benefit 3

You Can Workout At Your Own Pace

Treadmills allows you to determine the pace, distance, and complexity of the workout based on your needs. This means that it doesn't matter if you are just beginning to exercise or if you have remained fit over the years. As your fitness level improves, you will be able to adjust your machine to go faster, to work on a steeper incline or program it to help you burn more fat and calories.

Benefit 4

You Can Lose Weight

Any form of exercise will help you lose weight, but you have to do it on a regular basis. An exercise program on a treadmill will allow you to workout no matter how bad the weather and you won't suffer painful joints when you are finished.

Because of this you can do more workouts and for a longer periods of time. This means that you will burn more fat and calories, resulting in more weight loss.

Benefit 5

You Can Do Your Workout In The Comfort And Safety Of Your Own Home

How many times have you put off a walk on your street because it was too hot, too cold, raining, snowing, sleeting or hailing. The walk wouldn't have been much fun, would it? When walking on your treadmill you can watch TV, talk on the phone, listen to audio books or enjoy your favorite music. You can remain cool if it's too hot, or you can remain warm if it's too cold and you won't come home soaking wet from an unexpected rain shower. From my point of view, this is the best benefit of all.

No matter where your are in your fitness program, beginner or accomplished athlete, you can get many benefits from walking on a treadmill. Men over 50 will be able to lose weight, develop and tone muscles in the legs and develop an improved energy level. From the comfort and safety of your home, you can proceed from the very basic level of fitness to a level that will make you proud of yourself and proud of your new body.

WEIGHT LOSS ROUTINE STEPS FOR MEN OVER 50 YEARS

Relatively at this stage the energy in the man is partially depleted but Weight loss for men over 50 can still be attained but it has to be very easy and natural methods to develop interest and consistency for the result. Nature at this stage really prefers less tasking methods of fat burning process to enhance continuity, keep him fit and at the same time assist him to appropriately loose weight very easily in a healthy manner. The best option here is the workout routines which is the most suitable process for 50 plus men to effectively loose weight at a very convenient and enjoyable pace.

As the first step-On commencement you will need to do a warm up for between 5-10minutes depending on your capability. This warm up can be done via running on treadmill or cycling for a reasonable period of time with little boxing rounds. Ensure it is not too strenuous to avoid negativity and where you cannot complete it at a stretch some seconds of rest in between.

After this and for the next two minutes on this second step undertake push ups for as many times as possible within the allotted period. Respect the timing to avoid premature tire out. Follow the process carefully and enjoy the fun.

Use of jump rope can now follow as the third step. Definitely this is more energy sapping and can trigger few but temporary pains in your shoulders but you expected to start on a light basis. Also, your lungs may hurt initially but it will come out soothing thereafter. Your metabolism is enhanced and lots of fats will be burn off.

Having completed the light basis in step three, you are expected to rest for thirty (30) seconds before embarking on this fourth step which is supposed to be more intensive and more energy sapping but really interesting with the jump rope. There may be difficulties at the initial stage but consistency will get you accustomed to the exercise.

In this fifth step, gently kneel down; exercise while on your knees backwards and forwards to heat up your back and shoulders in a most gentle manner. Do this for like 1-2 minutes or more depending on your ability. Fat is gradually burnt in the process while you enjoy the processes.

As your body is gradually worked upon now you can now grab 10 or 15lbs dumbbells and continuously press the dumbbell to work out your shoulders for adequate flexibility.

Lastly on this step 7 you will make use of jump rope again in a more intensive manner that is higher than that of stage 4 to burn off the fat speedily. But care must be taken at this stage to ensure that you recognize your limit in order to know the appropriate time to stop.

Since we are talking of men over 50 here, I must warn that despite the simplistic nature of this routine you are expected to review your health status in order to pick the appropriate work outs that will not end up creating more problems to your health. If you are hypertensive or high in cholesterol level, you need to watch it and elect a suitable workout to achieve your objective.

MY DIETARY SUPPLEMENTS FOR MEN OVER 50 WANTING BETTER HEALTH

Are you taking a daily multivitamin? You don't get a pass on this one, supplementing daily with a good multivitamin is an absolute requirement for masters men over 50. Many items on my personal supplementation list are optional for many, but not the multi-vite, the holy grail of nutritional supplementation.

In fact, the only real debate of merit on multivitamins is what blend of nutrients andhow much of the recommended daily allowance (RDA) of each one should be taken.

Okay, so let's say up to this point you've totally missed the boat on multivitamins - why are multivitamins critical to the daily nutritional needs of men over 50? Without turning this into a science course the basics are as follow:

1. We don't get the essential nutrients in our daily diets. By and large, the typical US diet is pretty crappy. The main culprit is processed foods that have been mangled beyond recognition to our bodies.

However, even "clean eating" of whole foods like meats, fruits, and vegetables can leave us short due to mass-production techniques requiring low-cost and distribution requirements of durability and long shelf life.

Unless you're growing or raising your own food (yea, right) or buying from trusted local producers, your foods are likely lacking in their full nutritional potential.

2. If you're watching your calories to maintain weight or losing weight (you should be) then you're on a limited calorie budget for the three main macronutrient categories of protein, carbohydrates, and fats.

Therefore, due to these calorie constraints, you have limited opportunity to ingest the nutrients your body needs. Multivitamins give us these nutrients without adding calories.

3. Working out vigorously adds nutritional requirements as your body is in a constant state of repair and building (we're going to assume you work out if not you need to! Know that vitamins and minerals are the substances your body is either made up of or must have to synthesize into what it's made up of.

You can't have a glass of water without water, likewise you can't have a body (or at least a properly functioning body) without nutrients. And the more physical demand you place on your body, the more your body needs it's basic life ingredients.

So the next question is where the real debate starts; what vitamins and minerals should the senior athlete ensure is in their daily multivitamin uptake and how much of the RDA should be consumed?

Really, the consensus and even the science on this subject is all over the board, but my personal philosophy is to err on the high side.

Why?

Simple - because of research shows much upside promise to larger doses of multivitamins vs. a very limited downside.

Contrarily, some researchers suggest that extremely high dosages of certain vitamins can address specific health problems. This too tend to be more suggestive than conclusive, but I do personally go much higher overall on vitamins C and B complex (more on that upcoming).

This is what I feel is right for me based on my personal mix of diet and physical demands. And what I have found over many years makes me fee and operate at my best, you should talk with your doctor about what's right for you as many medical conditions, especially in senior men, may dictate special re☐uirements.

But I can tell you that personally, my overall approach to health, fitness and wellbeing includes mega doses, and that at 53 I feel as good as at any time in my life and get sick less than ever before.

PROMOTES HEALTHY AGING AND ACTIVITY WHILE COMBATING CHRONIC DISEASE

Weight loss for men over 50 requires a new approach over what worked in earlier years but is well worth the effort to master as it brings added benefits beyond a trim waistline including:

- Promotes healthy aging
- Increases productivity
- Combats chronic disease

As we age we lose muscle mass that is replaced with fat. Several things contribute to this and it's accepted as "normal" when nothing could be further from the truth. It is a process completely within our control.

As men, we produce testosterone and as we age the body slows production, assuming it isn't needed like it was when we were on the prowl for food and a mate or providing for our family. This results in a loss of lean muscle mass.

When we lose lean muscle mass our RMR-Resting Metabolic Rate-slows because lean muscle requires more energy to maintain than other tissue. While all these changes are taking place in our bodies there are a couple of things that are not changing:

The kind of food we eat and the portions we serve ourselves.

As we age our caloric requirements decrease as our RMS decreases roughly ½ percent per year. By default our caloric intake should also decrease but we rarely make that adjustment.

Healthy activity is common now for men over 50, If you don't already have a regular program of activity, then you should pursue it.

Weight Loss Promotes Healthy Aging

Excessive body fat promotes a number of conditions that diminish the quality of life in latter years. Proper attention to calorie intake and nutrition can have a positive effect on:

- Blood pressure
- Blood Sugar
- Memory
- Cholesterol Levels

- Life Span

- Weight Loss Promotes Increased Activity

As our weight and body fat percentage creeps up, it limits our activity. Reversing weight gain will have a positive effect in several areas:

- Increased Mobility

- Increased Energy

- Clearer Thought Processes

- Fewer "Sick" Days

- Weight Loss Combats Chronic Disease

There is ample, iron-clad evidence that overweight and obesity is directly related to chronic diseases like:

Coronary heart disease

Type 2 diabetes

Cancers, such as endometrial, breast, and colon

High blood pressure (hypertension)

High total cholesterol or high levels of triglycerides

Stroke

Liver and gallbladder disease

Sleep apnea and respiratory problems

Degeneration of cartilage and underlying bone within a joint

Reproductive health complications

Weight loss for men after 50 is one of the surest, easiest and least expensive ways to promote a high quality of life. It's not as easy as losing weight when younger and often discourages those who try. Knowing that the rules have changed and how to navigate your way will put you back in control.

CHAPTER TWO

NUTRITION AND ADEQUATE PROTEIN INTAKE FOR WEIGHT LOSS FOR MEN OVER 50

As men age weight loss becomes a challenge and it's especially tough for men over 50. Changes in our bodies reduce lean muscle mass and lower our RMR-Resting Metabolic Rate-causing an accumulation of fat.

This change is gradual and may not even register on the scale or tape measure right away. But the time clothing begins to tighten up and larger numbers register on the scale the process is already well on its way.

This onset of weight gain brings a predictable series of symptoms that will eventually develop into one or more chronic diseases. It is possible to reverse this weight gain with proper nutrition and close attention to protein intake.

Healthy activity and balanced nutrition, along with portion control, are keys to reverse weight gain for men over 50.

The purpose of this chapter is to explain why protein is important for weight loss in men over 50 and why so many of us miss the mark.

Protein is a building block of the body. Not just muscle, but connective tissues and organs all depend on a supply of protein in order to maintain themselves. When we don't get enough protein then the body goes after protein from stores in muscles. For men over 50 this means that not only are they losing lean muscle mass to the natural processes that come with aging, but they are losing lean muscle mass as a result of poor nutrition as well.

Our modern diet does not promote adequate protein consumption and often what protein we do eat is accompanied by unhealthy fat levels or carbohydrates that the body converts to fat.

Most men need between 150-180 grams of protein on a daily basis yet most get around one half of that amount. A body composition analysis will help you figure your personal protein requirements. Knowing your numbers will make it possible to map out a effective nutrition plan.

We can get protein from two sources.

Animal protein including red meats, poultry and fish are legitimate sources. One of the challenges of turning to these protein sources is the fat that may accompany them. Fatty red meats or poultry and fish prepared with heavy oils or sauces or breaded and fried are poor choices.

Dairy is also a source of animal protein. Milk, eggs, yogurt, cheese and other dairy staples are all good examples and fat is still a concern.

When turning to animal protein sources go for lean cuts of red meat-these often need marinating or slow cooking for tenderness-and prepare poultry and fish without excessive fats by baking or broiling.

Beans are an excellent source of protein as are a number of other vegetables. Plus these sources of vegetable protein also offer the added benefit of fiber.

Another popular source of non-animal protein are soy and whey protein. These send themselves to being added to other foods to boost protein content and to "protein shakes" as meal replacements.

The ideal balance is half of protein requirements from animal sources and half from vegetable sources.

For men over 50 the best approach is to calculate caloric requirements and build a healthy meal plan around those numbers. Getting the proper amount of balanced, healthy protein will support creation of lean muscle mass reverse weight gain or maintain healthy weight and tone.

MUSCLE BUILDING FOR MEN - ADVICE AND TIPS

If you are one of the senior men, it is a great news for you. You can build muscles from now with full confidence and therefore do not have to remain scared of the possible outcome. This has come out from a recent survey, and hence you should start from this moment. This is a great way that will make you retain your own vitality and hence you will look younger than your contemporaries. Isn't this great? On the other hand, you will remain healthy and also more confident than ever before. So try to follow a healthy workout always.

Now one may enquire any form of special training for senior men. This is the answer for them. There is no type of training that should be practiced only by the seniors. On the contrary, one should follow the general techniques but with verve. You must have the vigor and also patience since development of muscles due to strength training takes time. What is more it can take more time due to the reason of age. But never lose hope since it is bound to happen. Well, it is always better for you to check your own level of endurance. This is important since for the full-blown age you may suffer from several heart related diseases. For this it is necessary to go the doctor beforehand. If you are proved fit, then you should contact the trainer in the gymnasium at the earliest. The trainer is the best person to enrich you with the priceless advices.

From the very beginning you must attend on the aspect of achieving muscle failure. Are you hearing this for the first time? For this you shall have to lift a good amount of weight and with sufficient strength. This effort of raising more weight will teat and make your muscles ineffective. But when they will be cured, you will find them as more strong. This is the fundamental principle. Well, you can also go for the other forms of strength training on condition that you are advised by your trainer. You should use dumbbells if you are over 50. To the experts the dumbbells seems to be best since it enables one to work on different muscles of the body and at the same time. This means you do not have to concentrate on only one part of the body at each time.

Not only on exercises but your concentration should be also on diets. This is essential and the perfect combination of these two assists you to gain more muscles. If you eat 2 heavy meals on each day make it 5 from now. These new forms of meals should be small in ⬜uantities but rich in qualities. You should concentrate in the intake of more fresh fruits, green vegetables and also animal foods loaded with protein. They help you to retain your fitness and also nourish your body.

They do provide the support whenever the muscles break down due to exercises and also recover them. But never overstrain yourself. It is detrimental to health.

If you are over 50 and you want to get involved in weight training, it is by NO means too late! You can turn your life around for the better, be in great shape, feel great and restore lost energy that you didn't even know you had. Exercising is the best thing you can do for your body and it is extremely beneficial. Weight training for men over 50 is the best route to take, because it helps work on every muscle in the body and not just one, like with sit ups or crunches where you are focusing on your abdomen mostly.

Some important things to know related to weight training for men over 50, are that it's vital to stay hydrated. You can have serious complications resulting from dehydration. All you have to do is drink water and then drink some more water. Do anything you can do avoid dehydration! Coffee, soda, tea, iced tea and most drinks are all diuretics which DEHYDRATE you! You thinks you're quenching your thirst when really you are making yourself more and more dehydrated from all the salt and other ingredients. You must drink the recommended eight full glasses of water per day and perhaps even a little more especially on days that you work out.

Diet is also one of the MOST important thing in weight training for men over 50 years old. Proteins, complex carbs, essential fats, lean meats, vegetables…these are all vital parts in gaining muscle mass and actually achieving satisfactory results. If you can get up off the couch and shut off the TV, you'll find that weight training isn't so bad after all. You builds new brain cells when you exercise as well as get great feelings from the flow of endorphins in your body.

CHAPTER THREE

WORKOUT FOR MEN OVER 50

Slim Down and Charge up with a Fat Burning Workout for Men over 50

Age 50 can and should be an exciting time in the life of any man. Often it's a time when your kids are growing up, you've established yourself in your job, and you're looking forward to some of the great adventures that are left in your life.

Sometimes getting to the other side of 50 also means that you're carrying along some extra baggage. It's the unwanted extra few pounds that clings stubbornly around your waist and jiggles when you move. It's one of the things about getting older that you really don't appreciate. It's the reason that many men are looking for fat burning workouts for men over 50.

It seems so simple, but as with many things, easier said than done. If you want to lose some of that extra baggage then take in fewer calories and burn up the ones that you are taking in.

One of the other issues that often times accompanies men as they age is the fact that their metabolism slows making it more difficult for them to burn the calories that they take in. A slower metabolism means that the fat burning furnace isn't working to full capacity.

So what do you need to do to get your furnace stoked to the point where it's ramping up its fat burning capabilities to maximum capacity? It's important to eat a well balanced meal and it's also important to combine that with a fat burning workout that can get the job done.

Weight training and speed work of some sort are a few excellent workouts to help you burn some of those extra pounds.

Weight training can involve free weights or machines or it can also involve body weight training programs. Body weight training is becoming more and more popular because it doesn't require any equipment and you don't need to go to a gym or make room in your house for weight equipment.

Speed training as in hill sprints, martial arts training, punching and kicking a heavy bag, and just generally increasing the speed of the movements that one does and taking less of a break in between your sets are great ideas to ramp up that metabolism and start the fat burning fire going at full blast.

One of the fat burning workouts for men over 50 that is continuing to grow and gather up followers is the Combat Endurance Training workout. Developed by a Special Forces captain this workout offers elements of cardiovascular fitness, core and upper body strength work, and flexibility. The workout can also be ramped up to any level that the individual desires to achieve the maximum fat burning results.

Life after 50 can and should be invigorating. You've earned your stripes. It's a good idea to move into your golden years with a high level of energy, strength, and powerful attitude.

Fitness For Men Over 50 - Workout Routines For Obese Men Aged 50 Plus to Burn Fat and Lose Weight

Fitness for men over 50 is extremely important. Due to aging, most people encounters different types of diseases like Diabetes and high blood pressure that can be dangerous for them. In order to stay disease free and fit, one should shed those extra fats from their body. Men over 50 should be more conscious about their health. They should regulate their sleeping and eating habits and maintain a healthy lifestyle. Most men at this perform fewer activities, hence their metabolism slows down.

In order to generate metabolisms, they should take up cardio workouts. These exercises help us to burn fat. Your body remains active due to more supply of blood and good blood circulation. Your overall health is affected by a good workout regimen. Nutrition also plays a pivotal role in order to lose weight. Eating fat burning diets like acai berry supplements can be a good idea. You can also undergo colon cleanse for removing those toxic substances.

Workout Routines For Obese Men Aged 50 Plus To Burn Fat And Lose Weight

. Men over 50 should carry out mild exercises such as brisk walking, jogging and hiking. Walking generates metabolism in your body to burn fat. In order to lose weight healthily, drinking water is equally important. Water consumption hydrates your body and keeps your digestive tract clean. It also maintains your body temperature.

. Another great workout for men over 50 is hiking. You can explore nature and its tranquil beauty by performing this cardio workout. It will help your body to burn fat.

. Yoga is the best way to shed those extra pounds. It not only helps your body for weight loss but also rejuvenates your mind, body, and spirit, which is extremely necessary to maintain the fitness for men

Get Lean Workouts for Men That Are Effective

While there are several get lean workouts for men, some lifestyle changes also need to be incorporated. This includes reducing calorie intake, eating lean meats, poultry, fish, fresh fruits and vegetables, and switching from coffee and aerated drinks to water. You can also supplement your exercise routine with some diet and fitness products to facilitate weight loss and build lean muscle mass. However, getting lean requires some amount of effort, perseverance and time. It does not occur overnight. Men who exercise regularly and change their lifestyle habits will notice a consistent improvement.

Strength Training

Out of all the get lean workouts for men, strength training perhaps is the most important. When you do strength training, it helps to build muscle mass and this, in turn, helps to boost metabolism. Once the metabolic rate increases, the body burns more calories. You should be looking to work out every major muscle group in the body on three consecutive days. Your exercise routine should concentrate on large muscles and joint exercises that are performed in a circuit. You should not rest between sets to keep your metabolic rate high. Look at leg extensions, ball squats, step lunges, ball curls, pull ups, dumbbell chest flies and barbell rows to help build lean muscle. Avoid heavy weights, as it, will bulk up your muscles. Look at using moderate weights and doing about 10 to 15 reps at the most.

Aerobic Training

Aerobic training is an excellent way to burn calories, and ranks high among get lean workouts for men. You can do this training nearly all days of the week, but if you are looking to manage your weight, you should be looking at doing aerobic training 5 days in a week. In these 5 days, make sure that you do 30 minutes of aerobic training right after your strength training routine. In the remaining two days, you should be looking to do the workout for about 40 minutes. You should be looking to use standing aerobic e□uipment, such as treadmill, stair stepper and elliptical trainer. You can also look at cycling and swimming to help you burn calories by boosting your metabolic rate.

Pilates

Although Pilates is not that good at burning calories and helping build large groups of muscles, it involves stretching and strengthening all major muscles in the body. As a result it gives the body and leaner and longer look. Pilates can help men improve their posture. When you stand up straight, it can make you appear slimmer than what you are.

Getting that perfect six pack abs is dreams come true for men. It is generally seen among men that although they are fit, they wouldn't be considered fully fit if they still possess a protruding belly line. Health conscious individuals are constantly looking for best ab workout for men to maintain a lean and trim figure. There are no quick fix ways to get rid of this stubborn abdominal fat. You surely need to work hard towards it.

Here are some seven basic rules that you need to know about the best ab workout for men.

Patience and determination are important factors for any weight loss program. Today physical appearance and fitness has become very important and for that you really need to work hard on your abs as men generally tend to pile on weight in this area. Some men have heredity or some genetic problem of piling weight in the abdomen area.

Excess body fat can cause severe health problems like diabetes, obesity, blood pressure, oedema etc.

Best ab workout for men is cardiovascular exercise like running jogging etc which can be done on the treadmill and also on the elliptical or in actual setting. These cardiovascular exercises like spinning, biking, riding, jogging, etc. increases body metabolism and with better metabolism fats are burnt faster. Some of the abdominal exercises like crunches; sit ups etc surely help in removing excess fat. You need to work out for 30 to 40 minutes for a minimum of five days a week to lose fat around your abdomen.

· For the effectiveness of the best ab workout for men you need to work on your diet along with proper exercise. The belly fat is very stubborn and you really need to work hard on it to lose it. You should avoid all kind of junk food including fried and high processed foods. Instead increase the intake of fruits and vegetables in the diet and drink plenty of water to keep your system hydrated. Avoid instant and semi cooked microwave food.Instead eat freshly cooked food and avoid soft drinks.

· Another important factor that you need to consider for the effectiveness of the system is that you should never starve yourself or keep long intervals of food. In fact starvation causes weakness and also reduces metabolism.

· You should eat frequently but eat healthy and eat fresh fruit, vegetables, juices, white meat etc that are low in calories.By creating a calorie deficit in the body combined with working out you will lose your belly flab.

The, best ab workout for men, is cardio, jogging and abdomen exercises and these when clubbed with proper weight training you can develop the perfect six/ eight pack abs which so much coveted by people all over the world. The abs workout can be very strenuous and need a lot of dedication but once you see results you will get incentive to work harder.

CHAPTER FOUR

CLEAN EATING WORKOUT NUTRITION PLAN FOR MEN OVER 50

The following fitness and diet tips can help motivate you to stay active and to fuel your body with the right diet plan.

Fitness routines - Keep them Varied for Motivation

There are numerous benefits to mixing up your workout routine "It's the key to stimulating different muscle groups and preventing boredom."

Your body can easily get used to same physical activities if done repetitively enough. Alternating activities and exercise routines keeps the body guessing with the result being that more calories have to be burned as it has to adapt.

Don't go it Alone

Getting a fitness partner is a great way of keeping you motivated to stick with your diet plan and exercise routine. Your exercise buddy can help you stay focused as well as supporting and motivating you while exercising, as well as providing an element of competition - especially if you are of similar abilities.

Always Read Nutrition Labels

Whole, natural and where appropriate, raw foods should always be chosen over processed or pre-packaged ones, but if you are going to have a commercially pre-made or processed meal or food product, always read the label.

It's important to do so to avoid sabotaging your healthy eating plan -as not only do processed foods contain unhealthy ingredients much of the time, (trans fats, preservatives) but they also contain numerous servings in the one package - sometimes three to four - so it's very easy to overeat.

Cooking - Keep it Clean and Lean

When preparing meals at home, bake, grill, steam or lightly sauté. These cleaners (using less trans fats) cooking methods are healthier than breading and deep-frying. The use of healthy fats such as olive or coconut oil rather than butter will help keep the cholesterol levels down. Another great tip is to be creative with spices and herbs - they will help to keep meals more interesting and appetizing.

Eating - Keep It Vibrant and Exciting

The last thing you want is for your healthy eating plan to go astray because of diet boredom. Just like you'd try different ways to cook and prepare meals, try eating different foods and using unusual ingredients.

To add to your lean protein and low-fat dairy options, there are loads of different exotic fruits, vegetables and other products available in supermarkets and food stores these days, and more than enough cookbooks and recipes online to give you new ideas to try.

Limiting yourself to a similar range of foods, even if they are healthy, is not only a risk for diet dullness, but may also restrict your body from getting certain essential vitamins and minerals.

Size Matters

While on the subject of food, eat healthy and eat well, but watch the portion sizes. It's very easy to dish up large portion sizes - especially if that's what you were used to. Some good tips are to get smaller plates and to eat more slowly, chewing your food a lot more than usual - up to 12 times - so you get to feel full without eating as much food.

You can weigh the portions out and count calories according to the diet you are following, but a good rule of thumb is to eat a portion of protein no larger than the palm of your hand - and some simple carbs (veg and salad) of the same amount.

Strength Training is A Must

Including strength (resistance) training into your fitness programme is a great way to add variety to exercising as well as building calorie-burning muscle. There are many other benefits too:

- Increased body metabolism

- Improved bone strength and density

- Body toning

- Increased lean body mass

- Better balance and co-ordination

Strength training core muscles improves your balance for better overall athletic performance, and reduces the risk of injuries and common aches like backache. You don't need to use weights to do strength training - you can use bodyweight exercises, exercise bands - or even exercise in water.

Get HIIT to Work for You

Add some regular High-Intensity Interval Training to your fitness programme. HIIT has many benefits to offer for fat loss. Compared to steady state cardio exercises (like jogging) it saves time and can be more fun and interesting because of the variations in intensity. It will definitely help you lose fat quicker than steady state cardio, but you really have to push yourself.

Together with strength training, using HIIT exercises ensures your body gets optimum fat burning capabilities by increasing its metabolism both during, and after workouts.

Stick With It

Even with the best intentions and willpower, most of us will fall off the rails of our weight loss programme at some point - sometimes more than once. This doesn't mean we should quit - we will come across hiccups, we just need to get back on the programme and carry on. Jumping back on as soon as possible is important however, as the longer we let it slide the more momentum we lose and we have to start again.

CHAPTER FIVE

MUSCLE BUILDING, FITNESS AND DIET MYTHS

MYTH 1 >>Weight Training Turns Men to women.

TRUTH: This myth is particularly common because men worry that lifting weights will bulk them up If you were to look at 1 pound of fat, and 1 pound of muscle side by side, you would notice how much smaller the muscle is even though it's the same weight.

Which blows another myth out of the water, muscle is heavier than fat 1lb of muscle will always weigh the same as 1lb of fat.

Meaning, the more muscle you have on your body, the less space you will take up.

Men can not bulk up using heavyweights. Yes, heavier weights build muscle and strength

If men aren't supposed to have muscles, why have them? The definition of "manly" differs from one individual to another, but we all have a different body structure. Some men have more feminine lines; others more androgynous. Wide hip bones and narrow shoulders are typical female shapes, but that doesn't mean an athletic woman is less feminine. Our society forms our ideals; you choose what you find attractive.

MYTH 2>>I can spot-reduce my problem areas

TRUTH: Spot-reduction is not possible unless you go for surgery. Without it, your body will draw fat from different regions at different rates depending on your genetic makeup. Instead of focusing on one area, spend your time doing full-body workouts that blast calories.

This is the same for six packs or flat belly.

You can do crunches till you pass out, and you still might not get a six-pack. Save yourself the wasted time and probable back pain -- the best way to get a six-pack involves making better dietary choices and doing high-intensity interval training.

Everybody is born with abdominal muscles. You just need to lose fat to make them stand out.

MYTH 3>>Carbs are the Enemy

TRUTH: The only way to lose the right amount of weight is by adopting a balanced diet that supports your goal, training with weights, and doing some cardio. Your program should include all of these aspects long enough to see a difference.

Diet, weights, and cardio-the holy trinity of fitness!

If you want to gain muscle, you're going to need carbs. If you take them out completely, you'll burn more body fat during training perhaps, but you can't keep it up for long. Carbs are fuel for intense workouts, fats are not.

The macronutrients needed for a well rounded nutritional program are carbs, protein and fat. All three of these are necessary and have important functions within the body. I am not going to go into complete detail here as a complete breakdown of macronutrients and their function is extremely lengthy and would be better suited in an article on nutrition which I will write at another time.

The best way to phrase this myth would be - Which carbs are you eating and when?" Whole grains, legumes, vegetables and minimally processed grains are all good examples of the carbs that you can eat frequently

MYTH 4>>Running Is the Only Way to Lose Weight

TRUTH: Your fitness success depends upon your goal. If you want to be able to run 10 miles without breaking a sweat, then yes, you'll have to run.

If your goal is fat loss or muscle gain, the most effective way to lose weight is to include both cardio and weights in your routine.

Weight training is what keeps us upright, aligned and strong. Raising, the arches of our feet, strengthening our pelvic floor, and keeping our head from falling forward are the ultimate goals in preventing our bodies from collapsing as we age. Weight training strengthens tendons and ligaments as well as creates good bone density. While cardio can help with bone density and is an essential part of keeping your heart strong; it doesn't keep your body in alignment and strengthen your key postural muscles. Keep the balance and be sure weight training and cardio are in your repertoire.

MYTH 5>>The best time to exercise is early in the morning.

TRUTH: Unless you are a professional athlete training two to three times a day, then there is no one best time to exercise.

The best time is the time that appeals to you and fits into your schedule.

Listening to your body and knowing when you perform the best will help you decide if, in fact, mornings, afternoons or evening workouts are your time of power. Energy and attitude are keys in having great workouts. So learn your body clock, and try to hit the gym when you feel the strongest.

MYTH 6>>No pain, no gain.

TRUTH: A sign of a good workout is results, not soreness. Some localized muscular soreness that dissipates over a couple of days can indicate that you worked hard. To increase muscle and develop endurance you may need to experience a slight level of discomfort, but that's not pain. "No pain, no gain" is no good when it comes to developing a lifelong fitness plan.

Soreness is inflammation and the chemical response to inflammation. The only yardstick by which you need to measure progress is that of your goal. Judge your workout by what happens during that workout.

MYTH 7>>The best way to lose weight is to drastically cut calories

TRUTH: Our bodies are smarter than we think, When we eat too little, our body believes that it's starving so our metabolism slows down and holds onto fat as a potential energy source.

When some people try diets more than 90 percent of all people who lose weight by dieting gain it back.

Dieting for a quick fix is different from changing your eating habits

Eating healthy means developing a new mind set. The real trick to losing weight is a lifelong pattern of moderate exercise.

MYTH 8>>If you want to lose fat, avoid fat

TRUTH: Fats are necessary to maintain healthy hormone levels and make use of vitamins. Without it, you'll create a terrible environment for muscle growth. Fats also help you regulate your appetite. A carb-and-protein-only diet can make any fat-loss or muscle-build goal almost impossible to reach.

Healthy fats, such as Avocados, nuts, peanut butter, olive oil are "clean" and can help you lose weight are an important part of your diet, but having even a 100 percent clean diet doesn't mean you'll lose weight. You can be overweight and eat nothing but "clean" food.

MYTH 9>>You Can Eat What You Want If You Train Hard

TRUTH: You can't out train a bad diet.To burn fat, you need to expend more calories than your body uses. You can't hope to sit around and eat hamburgers all day and expect a few sessions a week to make you thinner. That's just silly.

MYTH 10>>The more you sweat, the more fat you lose

TRUTH: Sweat has nothing to do with intensity; it's your body's way of getting rid of heat. Fat is oxidized inside your body, and it is not going to vaporize because of you're sweating!

MYTH 11>> Fruit is a healthy snack that can't make you fat

TRUTH: We eat food because it gives us nutrients and fuel, but any kind of food, no matter how healthy, can make you gain weight. The fruit has a lot of easily accessible carbs. When you provide your body with easily accessible carbs, you're basically telling it to stop burning body fat for fuel. Also, fruit's sugar is mainly fructose, which is stored in the liver instead of in the muscles. It's also true that filling yourself with high-calorie fruit means you won't achieve your fat-loss goal.

Vegetables have more minerals, vitamins, and even more anti-cancer properties than fruit. The difference between the two food groups is the calorie content. In general, vegetables have fewer calories than fruit.

MYTH 12>> You can't gain muscle after 40

TRUTH: Age does bring wear and tear, but at 40 you're still a training baby unless you've been a competitive professional athlete since you were a teenager. The reason metabolism slows down as we get older is a combination of lower hormone levels and less athletic activity. You can build muscle at any age. As long as you're challenging your muscles and feeding them the proper nutrients, your body will respond. As you age, building muscle gets more challenging.

CHAPTER SIX

WEIGHTLIFTING AND EGO IN YOUR 50'S AND BEYOND

When it comes to weightlifting and exercise, ego has created a true dichotomy for those in their 50's and beyond. From commercial gyms and marathons to sports arenas and baseball diamonds you'll find older athletes of all ages, but then you'll meet just as many or more people in their 50's, and 60's who can only truly be referred to as 'old.' So what's the difference between these two groups and why is the gulf widening between 'boomers' and 'zoomers'?

The biggest difference is lifestyle, and lifestyle is a choice. And that choice is often based entirely on ego - how you see yourself. If you choose to judge yourself by financial success, you've probably made that your focus for most of your adult life, concentrating on making money and getting ahead, leaving little room for health, family time and outside hobbies. If you picture yourself as a parent and grandparent first, you're probably a nourisher who dotes on their kids and grandkids, even though it's meant a little less materialistic gain and probably carrying some extra poundage around each day. If you've always seen yourself as healthy and energetic, you've most likely been more careful to maintain healthy nutrition and been lifting weights, doing yoga or Zumba and/or been out running regularly.

And that's where the divide comes from - the lifestyle you've chosen up to this point. For most people, by the time you're in your 50's and 60's you've already experienced the illnesses, suffering and deaths of loved ones or even those you've grown up with. Staying in great shape, weightlifting, exercising and eating right food wouldn't have prevented all of those deaths. But how many might have avoided or at least survived those strokes, heart attacks and other fatalities if they'd been strong, healthy and carrying around the right weight for their frames, being neither underweight or overweight?

Look at what doctors and researchers say about diabetes, heart attacks and the like - over and over you've seen their advice to exercise to reduce the risks and severity. Look at seniors who has had bad falls - those that can cause a broken hip or pelvis, for example. Many never fully recover and pass within a couple of years, while stronger, healthier people heal fairly quickly and go back to their active life. And how many of today's diseases that plague older segments of the population come from a lifetime - or even a few years - of poor nutrition?

Even if you ignore the life-threatening situations and conditions, compare the daily lives of the two groups. Modern day life is filled with stress and that has a major effect on both mind and body - but it affects healthy people to a lesser degree as their minds and bodies are much stronger. How's your energy level? Are you too tired to get everything done and still go out in the evening? Or do you bounce out of bed when you get up and still love going out to the theater or a game and then out with friends for a late dinner afterward?

The bad news is you're where you are based on the choices you've made - and that's ego. The good news is you can rein in that ego, put some self-discipline into action and change the segment you're in. Because of the cumulative effect of your lifestyle to this point, the older you are the more imperative it is that you speak to your doctor and discuss what issues you need to consider as you change your diet and exercise level. Not the usual generic concerns, but what YOU, with YOUR history and in YOUR current condition, need to be aware of. In most cases, if you tell them you're serious about getting back in shape you'll get a hearty "Go for it!" from a very surprised medical professional - your history to date most likely didn't have them expecting you to suddenly value your health and wellness!

Here are the two biggest decisions you're facing:

1) What are your health & fitness goals?; and

2) Where should you start, given your current condition and age?

Let's start with the goals. If you're just into your fifties and haven't been keeping in great shape up til now, you'll need to watch your ego again. Men, you don't need, or even have any use for those big bulging muscles you once either had or envied.

What you want is a body that's capable of doing whatever you want to do, having the strength to do it and the energy to not only do that, but then continue merrily on with the rest of your exciting day, right? Oh, and waking up without all the aches and pains might be preferable too, yes? Being able to breathe after a 10k run at least as easily as you can today after climbing a single set of stairs? Another favorite of people in their 50's, 60's and beyond is being able to lay down at night and drift off to sleep quickly, then stay asleep long enough to wake up refreshed, energetic and ready to take on the world the next day. Put all those together and does that sound like something worth chasing and achieving? Great!

But while almost everyone in the 50's, 60's and beyond will agree with your goals, things vary greatly when it comes to where to begin. This is the most important aspect of getting strong and fits in your 50's, 60's and even your 90's and 100's, so give it considerable thought. You dont want to get hurt and end up in hospital - and that can happen to teens and twenty-somethings too if they start off wrong.

Contrary to what you might think, your age is not a big factor in this. A Canadian man was still running marathons at 100 years of age, and the oldest person to complete the grueling Iron Man Triathlon was an 84-year-old woman.

What does matter is your current state of health and how long it's been since you exercised regularly. If you've always stayed active and at or near your ideal weight, you can probably improve your nutrition and start lifting weights right from the get-go - just start light and build from there. If you've been retired for a few decades and spend most of your day dozing in your chair in front of the television, as long as your doctor approves of it start by walking a bit further each day. If you've got arthritis in your knees and hips and can only walk 100 steps, do it. Then tomorrow walk 101 steps. The next day 102 steps. And clean up your diet right away, since your ailments, don't affect your ability that way.

However, if you're morbidly obese at any age, start with diet modification. Replace the simple carbs and refined sugars in your daily meals with brown rice or yams, vegetables like broccoli and spinach and apples - all in reasonable moderation, of course. Work with your doctor to keep you on track and monitor your blood sugars and blood pressure, and once your weight has started to drop get your doctor's OK and start a walking regimen. Start with a shorter walk, going just farther than you've normally been doing each day to date, then build on that distance. Before too long you'll be able to lift weights too. Weightlifting helps two ways - the calories you burn while weightlifting and the new muscle you put on, muscle that burns calories 24/7.

Your goals in the gym, whether you're 50, 70, 90 or 110 should be improved strength, flexibility, stamina, and balance. Don't let a personal trainer or some gym rat tell you you need to stick to exercise machines to keep you 'safe' - using free weights that are the right weight for you and doing the big compound exercises with proper form will keep you safe. Avoid the urge to go too heavy, but don't let fear hold you back either. Start with a weight somewhat lighter than you think appropriate and increase it as time goes on. Hopefully over the years you've learned some patience, so starting lighter and working your way up to where you think you should start shouldn't be an issue. Wait til you see how you feel 2 or 3 days after the workout before deciding if the weight can be increased, and even then keep each increase small - fitness is a lifestyle, not a race.

While your body will still react like a teenager's in that it will build muscle and strength if you're lifting weights and eating right, it will take longer to recover between workouts, at least til you're back in fit condition. So start by planning two full-body workouts a week, on Monday and Thursday, Tuesday and Friday or Monday and Friday. At first, if you're still sore or stiff from your last workout, skip this workout. You won't get the same progress from just one workout that week, but you will keep from backsliding and losing any hard-won gains - and you'll be back to your 2 workouts a week in no time. A few months down the road you'll have the energy and strength to kick it up to three workouts a week but for the first few months stick to just twice. You'll know when to add in that third workout a week - your body will tell you.

None of this has to cost a lot - healthy nutrition is cheaper than fast-food outlets, and you can get started working out with a single pair of dumbbells and grow from there if need be. Look for results, not excuses. You're where you are through the choices you've made, and you can get to where you want to be by changing those choices and showing a little self-discipline and intestinal fortitude. Don't let your ego hold you prisoner any longer - start eating right and weightlifting intelligently and get back to truly enjoying an active and energetic life!

CHAPTER SEVEN

WORKOUT PLAN FOR MEN OVER 50

Great Tips On Work Out Plans for Men

Work out plans for men should incorporate both cardiovascular and strength training. What equipment is used, where the workout occurs and what exercises constitute the session are individual choices are not crucial to the effectiveness it. Everybody has access to different training equipment and has his preferred exercises for each muscle group. What is important is that the workout includes the six primary movements which form natural body moves and encourage a full range of motion. These movements are: squat, lunge, lift, push, pull and twist. Any program should include activities which involve these basic movements. Professionals suggest a weekly exercise routine which incorporates cardiovascular and strength training.

Work out goals are to add body tone and definition, while still including the significant health benefits of cardiovascular exercise. Exercise experts have developed simple, three-day work out plans for men that will help attain strength, power, and cardiovascular health. In a three-day plan, day one would focus on a muscle group or groups and cardiovascular exercise. This would be followed by a day of rest. This is vital for optimum results and also to avoid injuries. The second day of exercise would then focus on a different group of muscle(s) and cardiovascular exercise. A day of rest would follow this. The third cycle would exercise a different muscle group(s) and cardiovascular activity.

Good work out plans for men are limited only by the exerciser's interests, research, fitness level and age. Typical exercises might include these muscle-building exercises: planks, lunges, horizontal leg raises, floor crunches, push-ups, chin-ups, jumping jacks, squats, wall stands, and twists. Cardiovascular activities might include: jogging, running, swimming, bike and exercise bike riding, jumping jacks and treadmill walking.

It is important that any program begin with a warm up to stretch and prepare muscles to work and a cool-down activity. As with the day of rest between exercise days, warm ups and cool downs are critical to avoiding injury and maximizing the benefits.

Variety in the specific exercises is also important. Variety ensures that different muscle groups are not being over-exercised and thus prone to injury while other muscles are being allowed to atrophy. Exercises which emphasize different muscle groups should form part of the training program. As well, the entire work out plan should be changed every two weeks or so.

This may seem obvious but in devising a work out plan it is important to ensure all muscles are being exercised and strengthened: abs, back, biceps, triceps, thighs, hips, chest and cardiovascular. Refraining from over-exercise is as vital as exercising. It is critical that the routine be based on convenience. The location: home, office, gym, outdoors, indoors is not of paramount importance when setting up a routine. But the program must fit into your lifestyle. Whether you're at home without access to a fitness center or on the road, a must be able to be done anywhere, anytime. Work out plans for men in particular that fit these important criteria leaves the exerciser with no excuses for slacking. This may also seem obvious but it is very helpful when the workout program is reasonably attainable and fun and the exerciser must be able to see results.

3 Tips for a Workout and Diet Plan for Men

Women are attracted to men who are strong and healthy; it's written in their genetic code. Instead of moping around and trying to fight nature, it pays off big time if you work with it to your advantage. Finding a workout and diet plan for men will work wonders for helping you regain your confidence in your body. By working out and eating right, you can get the body that all of the ladies will be drooling over. Below are three tips that will help you formulate a workout and diet plan for men that will get you the body you want.

Tip 1 - Body Targeting

When you start any workout and diet plan for men, it will benefit you to target a specific part of your body that you want to change. This is because most workouts are designed to target a specific area of the body, such as the chest or arms or even the legs. By focusing on one area at a time, you will notice results quicker. Not only will result come quicker, but can you imagine how long your workout would have to be if you wanted to maximize the effectiveness on every part of your body at once? It would take forever, so what's most likely to happen is that you'd work out each part of your body minimally and wouldn't get any results at all.

Tip 2 - Resting Is Important

One of the biggest mistakes made by people on a workout and diet plan for men is that they neglect to factor in rest times. Believe it or not, you aren't really a super hero. You need time to rest between workouts so that your body can heal. That is what actually builds muscle. When you work out, tiny fibers in your muscles actually tear, and it is the healing of these tears that builds up your muscle. Rest for at least a day after every workout session, and two days if you are just starting.

Tip 3 - Eating Right

Plenty of protein in the diet will help you build muscles faster than anything else. Chicken, turkey, fish, eggs, and even some types of vegetables are great sources of protein. Eat six meals spaced evenly throughout the day instead of three. This will speed up your metabolism so that you can burn fat while you build muscle. After all, you need to burn fat at the same time; otherwise, your muscles won't show through the inevitable layer of fat covering them. Drinking plenty of water will help you stay hydrated and heal faster after workouts.

By following these three tips, a workout and diet plan for men are going to come naturally to you. By eating right, targeting specific areas of your body, and remembering to rest after each workout, you can build the body you have always wanted. You will attract the women you have always wanted to attract and in the process, you will feel healthier and stronger than you have ever felt in your life.

Weight Loss Secrets For Men Over 50

High blood pressure, high cholesterol, you're a heart attack waiting to happen-whatever the doctor told you-you know you've got to get those pounds off, pronto! You want to know--are there any weight loss secrets for men over 50?

Yes, you want, and really need to experience rapid weight loss because your life depends on it. You want that top-of-the-world feeling and lots of confidence. You're overweight and you're already in the high-risk category of developing diabetes and high blood pressure.

This is why thousands of men search for an easy way to slim down. But should you adopt a rapid weight loss regimen? Before you start joining any dieting programs, check with your doctor first, and you've already done that.

To lose weight effectively, pay attention to what you eat, how you eat, your behavior and your activity level.

Here are nine tips for successful weight loss:

1. Adopt a diet plan that suits to your tastes and budget. You don't have to sign up for those weight loss programs that provide the food for you. In fact, you'd be better served to learn how to prepare the food yourself.

2. Exercise at least 15 minutes a day, such as brisk walking, running, swimming or dancing. Even doing chores around the house such as sweeping, vacuuming and mopping the floor (your wife would love that!) and washing the car are considered as exercises. Line dancing is also one of the best and more exciting ways to lose those calories! Just chooses the ones you'd be more apt to do on a consistent basis. Consistency is key!

3. Set realistic goals. Baby steps help you reach your goals more effectively. Start with small changes in your food. Make bigger changes as you go along. Discipline and a positive mind-set yield that can-do spirit!

4. Listen to your body. Try different exercises or diet plans to see which suits your body best. For example, your body may not be able to take the rigors of aerobic workouts. It is comfortable with brisk walking. Hence, brisk walking may be more suitable. Work with your body, not against it, to see faster results.

5. Include more fiber in your diet. It makes you feel full longer. Fiber also aids digestion and elimination.

6. Keep away from fried and deep-fried foods. These are practically dripping with fat. Although fish and chicken appear leaner than beef, these white meats contain more fat than when fried than beef does. Go for grilled or broiled food as this contains less fat after cooking. Don't, however, avoid fat completely. Just use more healthy fat. Extra virgin olive oil is one of the good ones. Still, be conservative in the amount you use.

7. Drink at least six to eight glasses of water a day to keep your body hydrated. It also helps your body to eliminate body wastes more effectively. This is easily accomplished and there are a number of ways to do it. Keep a bottle of water near your workstation and remind yourself to drink a gulp or two periodically. Keep 5-oz paper cups near the water source and make yourself get up and drink two cups every once in a while. Keep a bottle of water in your car.

8. Last, but the most important: RESOLVE TO MAKE THIS YOUR NEW LIFESTYLE!! Rapid weight loss programs, crash diets, and drastic exercises just bring about yo-yo weight loss creating more health problems than you resolve. Oftentimes, you put more weight back on than you ever took off. Over time, you could become obese.

9. Let's add one more-join a support group for encouragement AND accountability.

CHAPTER EIGHT

FASTEST WAY TO GAIN MUSCLE

Your body is designed and hardwired to put on muscle and burn fat. All you have to do is follow the steps and your body has to build lean muscle. There are 3 things to keep in mind when trying to gain muscle fast: Eating enough, Training enough, and Sleeping enough.

Eating enough is the fastest way to gain muscle

One of the most common problems you see in gym-goers today is not eating enough. You knows the guys, the ones that look the same every single month. They are not feeding their body what it needs to grow. It's like pimping out your car without even putting gas in it!

You needs about 1 gram of protein/pound of body weight in order to build muscle mass. You also need carbohydrates to fuel your body. Aim for 400 grams carbohydrates a day when bulking. Also, try to consume good fats such as peanut or almond butter. A great way to get your calories in is a modified protein shake. Here's my own recipe:

- 1 cup of oats
- 4 tablespoons of peanut butter
- 1 banana
- 2 cups of white whole milk
- 2 cups of chocolate whole milk
- 1 serving protein powder

1 shake has 1830 calories, 83 grams of protein, over 200 good carbohydrates, and healthy fats your body needs! Simply combine all the ingredients in a blender for a really easy way to meet your daily macro-nutrient goals.

Training enough is crucial and one of the fastest ways to gain muscle

You have to really be in tune with your body to understand how to train effectively. If you are a beginner, you should train 3 days a week. If you are intermediate or advanced and have a training split, you have to know how to strategically position your rest days. This is important because it allows your body to get the recuperation it needs (which is actually when muscle is being created).

Recently, I noticed that my lifts were starting to go down in the gym. It was odd because I was eating enough good food to gain weight. Through having a mind-muscle connection I was able to stop and decide that the best thing would be to take a couple days off. It was this insight that allowed me to come back to the gym even stronger. More importantly, it allowed me to keep progressing.

Progression is the single-most important thing to building muscle. You can measure your progression by increasing weight while staying in the hypertrophy repetition range (8-12 reps). By viewing it this way, you can be positive that you have grown if you have also increased the weight used during a particular exercise.

Finally, getting enough sleep is mandatory when you find the fastest ways to gain muscle

Sleep is when your body is actually building itself back up after workouts. If you can dial in your training and nutrition with healthy sleep patterns, your gains will skyrocket. The key here is making sure to always listen to your body. If you try to follow a plan without tailoring it to your body, you would get worn down and stop progressing.

Natural sleep aids such as melatonin can help cultivate deep sleep. However, no sleep aid is as good as a nutritional diet and a workout plan that fits your fitness level. Focus on these 3 things to accelerate your muscle gains and reach a better you!

Where to start when looking to build muscle can be confusing. There are many different routines for men out there, but not all of them are good. In this article, I will be showing you some essential components to any workout program. These key factors need to be in the routine if you want to get the best results possible.

Workout programs that contain individualized workouts.

This is the very first thing that needs to be considered when looking at a good muscle building routine. Many workout routines contain a one size fits all workout. The workout is meant to be done by everyone, and that also means that everyone is supposed to get the same results from the program. Everyone is unique in their own way with things like different body types, metabolisms, heights, and weights. It is absurd to think that one single workout will provide the same results to the people that do the workout. A good system will provide individualized workouts based on your different measurements and needs.

Programs that contain individualized nutrition.

This is the next key factor to consider when determining a good muscle building routine from a bad one. Nutrition is very important when it comes to building lean muscle. It is important that a routine does not come with a generic meal plan that everyone is supposed to be able to follow. Things like total calories, protein, carbs, and fat all need to be based around the individual's specific needs. It will also be very boring to be eating the same things over and over again. Sound nutritional programs will be individualized and will also provide you with many options for what to eat so that boredom never becomes an issue.

Simplicity and ease of use.

The final key to a smart and effective workout is that the routine is easy to get started. If a program comes with a two hundred page book to read before you are allowed to get started, then it is unlikely that you will do the program. Also if the muscle building rountine is just plain confusing and unorganized, then it, will be very hard to know where to start at. Any good routine will come with a quick start guide to help you know what exactly you need to do in order to get started. The guide also won't be hard to read, long, or complicated either.

The best thing that you can do is get started working out right away! No matter how good any program is, no program can help with laziness. At the end of the day you must put in the work and dedication and the results will soon follow assuming you are following a good muscle building routine. Use the three factors described above to help determine if a certain workout is right for you. Once you have decided on one, the only thing left is to actually do the program and start to get the results that you have always desired.

It is not clear why, but the majority of men want a well-developed, muscular chest and ladies according to to studies and polls are pleased with this muscle building priority. Strong, proportional and large pectoral muscles are often seen in subconscious level as a primeval demonstration of strength and confidence. Of course chest still has a huge physiological, functional and visual value. So what to do then? Head to the nearest gym? Maybe. However, there are chest exercises for men, which costs nothing and can give impressive results (women can use this same method, but they may want to adjust the intensity).

His Excellency Push-up.

While some people feel that this humble exercise is good only for secondary and high schools, in reality push-ups can beat some very trained athletes. Be sure, it IS possible to use push-ups to gain muscle mass or strength, if you know how to progressively increase load and intensity. And no, I am not talking about stuffing a backpack with heavy books while doing gazillions of push-ups...

Progressive training.

Whether you train for maximum size, strength or muscular endurance, it is important to know how to increase the intensity of the exercise. These are the basic steps.

1. Beginners perform push-up with their hands on a stable table or chair. Yes, it doesn't look impressive yet. The key is to do it with a flawless technique.

2. Now start to do push-ups with your hands and knees on the floor. This is already targeting your pecs and triceps quiet seriously.

3. Classic push-ups. Place hands wider and push a bit elbows away from torso to work your chest more.

4. Place a small stool under foot and do push-ups. If it's too hard position, you can even place just couple of phone books; later use high chair. These decline push-ups train the upper part of the pectoral muscle.

5. With both feet on the floor, you start to place your arms in different asymmetrical positions to put the lion's share of weight on one of the arms. Always mirror every arm position, with train both arms e☐ually

6. Begin to place small books under one arm and perform push-ups. Then place books under other hand and exercise other side. Develop your push-ups to the level where you can make a push up with one hand on at least nine inch high support.

7. Replace the solid support of one hand to an unstable one like basketball or kettleball.

8. Start to gradually place the support farther away from center of your body when doing your push-ups.

9. Introduce one-arm push-ups into your routine.

10. Place both feet on a solid stool and perform one-arm push-ups. You can start to experiment with one-arm, one(opposite)-leg push-ups.

CHAPTER NINE

TIPS ON DIET AND EXERCISE FOR MEN

Diet and exercise for men are the two things you need to pay attention to for a healthy and fit body. The body needs to be conditioned with the right type of exercising, along with being filled with the right nutrition. In this article, I will give you some tops to eating right and exercising in the correct way. Diet and exercise for men is extremely important, and if you would like to start looking better, these tips are going to help you out in the long run.

Tips on Diet and Exercise For Men

- Always Eat Protein-Filled Foods and Good Carbs

Eating foods that are high in protein and good carbs such as vegetables is the right way to go. This is basically the cave man diet; if you can pick it or kill it, you can eat it. But if it's combined, mixed and mashed up and then dehydrated and put in a box with lots of sugar and chemicals then stay the heck away from it. It will do you more harm than good. And speaking of good, I know most of it tastes real good but get over it. Eat LEAN MEAT, and fresh vegetables and fruits.

Once you detoxify from all of the crap added to the food chain you will begin to have more energy and your natural metabolism will help you lose weight and feel better.

- Protein Shakes

If you skip one of your meals, you could supplement it with a nice protein shake. Protein shakes have a lot of healthy nutrients for your body. Shakes can be gulped down throughout your workouts, before the workouts, and after the workouts. Protein shakes can be the perfect thing to take if you lack extra energy, NOT the energy drinks with tons of caffeine that are advertised, so make sure that you add them to your diet.

- Eat After You Workout

After you workout, you will find that your body needs a lot of food to help your body recover. You have actually lost many calories and weight from your workout, and when you eat after you workout, you actually help your body recover. The recovery period after a workout is the most important time to avoid fatigue and pain throughout the body and eating after your workout is the key. To help you recover quicker, drink anything with protein inside of it, or better yet try a protein shake.

- Lifting Free Weights

If you start a weight lifting program, you would add muscle and reduce fat. Doing a 20 to 30 minute lifting program with seven to ten different exercises every other day is a great way to start. Take it slow and begin with low weight and add more when you can perform at least three sets of fifteen repetitions of each exercise with no straining.

Building your workout routine slowly and changing your exercises up, so you don't burn out one muscle group is important. A good way is to split your routine into upper body on the one day and lower body the next day you lift with a rest day in between. You can do a short but intense cardio workout on your rest day. I like to lift three days a week and do cardio on the two days in between and then take two days off completely to allow muscle to heal and grow.

- Correct Form

If there was one aspect that many guys forgets, it would be to exercise and lift weights in the right form. The way that you workout is vital to ensure that you workout with the best possible form. I highly suggest that you workout effectively by paying attention to what you do while you workout.

- Avoid "Just Running" For Cardio

You may think that running is important, but it can be rough on your joints and can cause injury that will prevent you from working out. Varying your cardio with jogging, swimming, biking and aerobics are great ways to get your cardio too. You also can do other sports also, such as basketball or volleyball or any highly aerobic sport.

-Consistency of Effort

Just keep in mind the tips above only work if you do them consistently. A good diet and weight training program is the best way to get healthy and to live a happier life. Take it day by day and week by week.

3 FAT LOSS RECIPES FOR MEN

Weight loss for men does not have to include starvation. In fact, eating healthy is the key ingredient to weight loss. Start with a healthy breakfast. This will not only help to curve food cravings throughout the day, it is one of the keys to success in weight loss.

Avoid the cereals and oats for breakfast and start with a meal such as an omelet. Omelets are high in protein, high in veggies and low in carbohydrates- which will help aid in losing fat.

Omelets are relatively simple to make simply start with:

Omelets:

Ingredients:

* 2 eggs

* 2 tablespoons whole milk

* 2 tablespoons butter

* Salt and pepper to taste

* Veggies: you can do a combination of veggies or just one. Suggestions include mixed peppers, baby spinach, Brussels sprouts and broccoli

* Meats: meat is optional but can include ground round, chicken ground slices, bacon, minced beef or tuna

* Cheese: cheese can include grated cheese, feta cheese, parmesan or Pecorino

* Spices: wonderful spices to spice up the omelet cayenne pepper, cumin and sea salt.

Break the eggs into a bowl and beat them. In a nonstick skillet, melt the butter. Once the butter is heated, pour in the eggs to the pan. Add the different ingredients and cook. When, the omelet is one on one side, fold the omelet in half and cook on each side.

Lunch:

Cottage Cheese. This is a great meal. Low in carbohydrates and high in protein. And, there is absolutely no preparation, just possibly spicing it up a little more.

Foods you might like to add to your meal include:
- Almonds
- Walnuts
- Cashews
- Raisins
- Peanut butter
- Sliced banana
- Pears
- Apples
- Berries
- Tuna

Dinner:

Macho Meatballs

Ingredients:

- 1 pound extra lean ground beef
- cup of crushed saltine crackers
- 1clove garlic
- 1 large onion diced
- 1 tablespoon whey powder
- 1 jar tomatoes sauce
- cup shredded mozzarella cheese

In a bowl, mix the meat, crackers, garlic onion and whey powder. Using your hands, for the mixture into round golf ball sized portions. Cook in a non cook skillet until they are done. Add the tomato sauce. Warm and serve. Sprinkle the mozzarella cheese over the top when serving. Makes four servings.

If you find yourself craving foods throughout the day, grab something nutritious. Carrot sticks and celery are excellent to snack on throughout the day and definitely help one with the energy and the nutrients the body needs for staying fit and healthy. Weight loss does not have to be a chore; it can be very accommodating.

If you are overweight and have been struggling to lose those unwanted pounds, the fact is that the foods you eat are likely one of the biggest culprits in your weight issue. So taking time to pick from among the available diet plans for men and putting the plan you choose into action is an important step toward taking control of your weight issue. Yet diet plans for men alone are not the only answer, and other changes must be made in your life, too. These are some changes that you will find can help you to lose your weight and keep it off once your diet is over.

Change Recipes: Whether you are the main cook in your life or your spouse is, you will want to make an effort to really analyze what you have been eating and compare it to the foods included in your diet plan. Many recipes that you currently follow may be altered slightly to accommodate your diet plan, and this is a great way to not just enjoy a nice transition into your diet now but also to stick with it for many months and years to come as a weight maintenance plan once those pounds are gone.

Water: Some diet plans for men sing the praises of water and others do not. You may think that you are drinking enough water every day, but you likely are not. Consider that water is not interchangeable for other liquids. Sure, water is used to make coffee, tea, sodas, and more, but these other drinks are loaded with ingredients that actually dehydrate you and pull water out of your cells, such as caffeine and sugar. Plus, sugary drinks are surely to be avoided on your diet plan, too. What's more, many times thirst is mistaken for hunger, and you may find that by drinking more water throughout the day, you cut down on the urge to snack.

Exercise: Enough cannot be said about the important of leading an active lifestyle. Now if you are severely overweight and currently lead a very sedentary lifestyle, the mere thought of lacing up your sneakers can make you exhausted. However, exercise should be included as a part of any diet plans for men. You will want to make an effort to get out of the house and at least go on a bike ride, a walk, or a slow jog for about 30 minutes per day. It doesn't matter what you do as long as your heart rate is elevated and you are moving. You will find that adding some strength training can improve your weight loss efforts, too, as building muscle helps you to burn fat. Something as simple as investing in some dumbbells and using them while you watch TV can do wonders for you.

As you can see, there truly is more to losing weight and keeping it off than simply following diet plans for men. Diet plans are a fabulous way to lose weight, and care should be taken to find the right one for you. However, you will also want to incorporate these changes into your lifestyle, too, if you want an easier time losing weight and keeping it off.

VITAMINS AND MINERALS FOR THE OVER 50'S

As promised, here is an over-view of the main essential vitamins and minerals, but, rather than take them in isolation it is better to take a good multi-vitamin and mineral tablet aimed specifically at the over 50s.

Vitamin

What it can do for you, for example -

Found in, for example -

Helpful Advice

A

Promotes growth, strong bones, healthy skin, hair, teeth, and gums. It Builds resistance to respiratory infections. Good for eyes, particularly night blindness.

Carrots, fish oils, eggs, green and yellow vegetables, milk and dairy products

10,000 iu is the average daily dose. Prolonged high doses can be bad for you as it can be stored in the body.

B

Helps to maintain a healthy nervous system, muscles and heart and energy. Good for stress and aids memory.

Whole-wheat, whole brown rice, oatmeal, bran, milk, liver, fish, vegetables, beef, pork, nuts, fruits.

It is a good idea to take all the various B vitamins in one B complex tablet. Smoking and alcohol can deplete the body of this vitamin.C

Aids in the prevention of the common cold, infections, helps repair body tissues, eg. helps healing after surgery.

Citrus fruits, green leafy vegetables, tomatoes, potatoes. NB. It is generally not a good idea to eat citrus fruits, eg oranges, grapefruits, etc. If you suffer from arthritis.

Helps the body absorb iron. Vit C works best when taken with calcium and magnesium. Vit C is excreted from the body quite quickly, so it is a good idea to take a time-release tablet. Smoking can destroy Vit C.

D

Works with calcium for strong bones and teeth

Acquired through sunlight, eating plenty of fish and fish oils, and dairy products

Dosages over 5,000 iu daily not recommended. Dark-skinned people is living in northern climates usually need to take additional Vit D.

E

Good for the skin and helps you to look younger. It helps healing of burns, and helps with fatigue.

Wheat germ, soya beans, broccoli, spinach and leafy greens, whole-grain cereals and eggs.

Iron tablets destroy the efficiency of Vit E if taken together - allow 8 hours between. Women over 50 and menopausal women should increase their Vit E intake.

MINERALS

Calcium

Essential for strong bones and healthy teeth

Milk, cheese, soyabeans, sardines, walnuts, sunflower seeds and green vegetables.

Calcium and iron are the two minerals often deficient in a woman's diet. Dolomite tablets are a natural form of calcium and magnesium

Iron

Necessary for the production of red blood corpuscles (haemoglobin). Prevents iron-deficiency anaemia and fatigue.

Red meat and offal, egg yolks, nut, beans, molasses, oatmeal

For normal adults the recommended amount is 10 - 18 mg, but before increasing the amount (perhaps because of fatigue, etc), it is better to consult your doctor. It is worth noting that ferrous sulphate, a form of iron that appears in many supplements, may destroy your Vit E: the chelated form of iron is preferable.

Magnesium

Necessary for the optimum functioning of nerves and muscles. Helps fight depression. Good for the heart.

Figs, nuts (in particular almonds), seeds, apples, grapefruit and apples.

People who suffer from cramp are often deficient in magnesium. Alcoholics are also usually deficient. Dolomite (a balanced formula of magnesium and calcium) is a good quality supplement.

Selenium

Works with Vitamin E and appears to slow down the aging process. Helps with energy.

Wheat germ, tuna fish, onions, broccoli, tomatoes, bran

Selenium is important to human nutrition. Because of intensive farming and food processing techniques, many of our foods are depleted of Selenium.

Zinc

Good for the immune system, muscle function, and blood and brain function. It can also help with healing.

Choice meats are such as steak and chops, wheat germ, pumpkin seeds, eggs.

Men should keep their zinc levels up, particularly if worried about prostrate problems. Zinc and manganese are thought to help ward of senility in the elderly.

REMEMBER: What you put into your body is what you get out of your body! So think of food as fuel and choose food from the chart above.

Sadly, cakes, biscuits, etc. are merely 'comfort' foods and not nourishing fuel for the body.

NOW HERE ARE A FEW MORE SUPPLEMENTS TO HELP YOU 'SPRING' INTO SPRING.

Co-enzyme 10 The body's 'spark-plug' for energy.

Ginkgo Biloba Helps maintain good circulation to the body's extremities (so good for those who suffer from cold hands and feet). Also improves blood supply to the brain and helps with poor memory.

Glucosamine Helps maintains connective tissues in the joints and is believed to stimulate cartilage growth and promote smooth functioning joints.

Echinacea Boosts the immune system - an aid in the prevention of colds and flu.

Garlic Also boosts the immune system and, importantly, has antiviral, antibacterial and antifungal properties.

Omega 3 fish oils. Benefits heart, circulation, joints and brain.

Evening Primrose Oil Good for the immune system and appearance of skin.

So all the above are a bonus for the over 50's.

HRT CAKE

Ingredients:

50 gr sunflower seeds, 50 gr pumpkin seeds, 50 gr linseeds,

50 gr sesame seeds, 50 gr almond flakes, 50 gr raisins.

100 gr cranberries, 150 gr chopped dried apricots,

2" stem ginger, chopped, ½ teaspoon nutmeg, ½ teaspoon cinnamon,

1 tablespoon malt extract, 3 tablespoons apple juice,

425 ml (approx) of soya milk (add more milk if necessary to make a soft dropping consistency).

Method:

Mix all the dry ingredients in a large mixing bowl.

Add the cranberries, apple juice and soya milk and stir well.

Leave to soak for approx ½ hour.

Pre-heat the oven to 190°C.

Line a loaf tin with baking paper and spoon mixture in.

Cook in pre-heated oven for approx 1¼ hrs.

When cooled, slice and store in freezer.

CHAPTER TEN

WHAT ARE THE NECESSARY THING TO CONSIDER FOR MEN OVER 50

Men over the age of 50 are still active and in their prime. But to maintain and prevent the onset of illness and ailments, men should consider these tips once they reach this age. Go for a physical exam annually. As your body ages, some physical symptoms are also seen. You can discuss these with your doctor. Seek advice on the treatment of minor ailments and steps on the prevention of other diseases such cancer, hypertension, diabetes, and heart disease. Included in the physical examination are routine blood tests, urine and stool tests, and physical tests like treadmill, ECG, and lung x-rays.

• Have your blood examined. For blood tests, you should test for cholesterol levels. This can help you determine if you are eating right and if you have healthy habits. This can help you prevent the onset of hypertension or heart disease. Smokers and diabetics usually have high cholesterol levels.

• Go for rectal and colon exam. Undergoing stool testing, colon testing, and rectal exam annually can be a great help in detecting the growth of polyps or cancer of the colon.

- Regularly visit your dentist. These regular oral examinations can help in the early detection of tooth decay, disease of the gums, or oral cancer. Those with unhealthy habits like smoking, chewing of tobacco, and poor oral hygiene run the risk of many dental problems. Some studies suggest that heart attack and stroke are closely associated with gum disease, so this is a serious matter.

- Have your eyes examined? The annual examination of your eyes is very important as this can detect problems with your vision such as glaucoma or the early onset of cataracts.

- Have your annual prostate examination. A prostate exam is a very important test for men of age 40 and above. This can help in detecting prostate cancer early, which can give you a high percentage of survival.

- Visit a psychotherapist. Not for anything else, men should visit a doctor to screen for depression. Your mental health is as important as your physical health. Talking to a doctor can help you with underlying depression or anxiety.

As with everything else, eating right along with having regular exercises are the most important ways to prevent diseases. Most importantly, these physical examinations and healthy practices can go a long way in early detection and the higher survival rate against diseases.

As we get older, obviously we change - our musculature, our desires, and our energy. We tend to get lazier than when younger. Though I think this is a society habit rather than an age habit. Here are some tips to maintain health and energy as we mature.

1) You lose muscle tone as you age, take up weight training, if you have never done it before - take advice and start slowly - but build back your muscle tone. You can easily do weight training into your 70's and 80's. Keep your body from falling literally down.

2) Get your weight down. If you are overweight, be brutal with yourself, get your weight down, slim down, don't carry that extra weight. When you were younger your body could take more punishment - be gracious with your frame and body now. Allow its spaces. So eat lean. Allow your heart to work less, be kind to your veins and arteries. Take away the physical stress on your organs. Get the weight off your bones and joints. Improve your muscle tone but avoid the fat.

3) Get your blood pressure under control. Heart attacks are lethal and have no warning signs - except blood

pressure. You can die at 40 or 80 of a heart attack, and their is no warning. Check, your blood pressure, get it within a healthy range. But unless critical - try to avoid drugs - use exercise diet and nutrition.

4) Eat less and eat healthier - your body and its systems don't process food as well as at twenty - give them leeway, treat them kindly. Moderation in all things. Cut out the obvious fat and sodium monsters.

5) Take vitamins. Vitamins and mineral tablets may not do much if your are slim and trim and on a healthy diet. But your body needs help in procuring a lot of things it had no problem with at twenty five Take a multivitamin - it won't hurt. Ideally a premium one (that is one that works as a food and is not just artificial vitamins in starch and sugar) One of the best is Nutrilite brand

6) For health - think nutrition first before prescription drugs. Prescription drugs are always a problem. They are emergency treatment- not lifestyle treatment. Glucosomine for joints, omega 3 for immune system and healthy heart. Garlic for cleansing and heart health. Ginseng for energy (be careful with good ginseng its ☐uite the booster).Coenzyme Q10 for energy replacement.

However with all supplements, please consult a knowledgeable health professional, who knows your lifestyle and body type.

7) Produce more joy than worry in your life. Make plans. Think you're old? Hey you could be dead tomorrow - or you could have another 50 years (your life so far, over again) Set a goal, get a desire, make plans. You are always happier on the way to a desire. It may be time to retire from the job - but life is rich and omnipresent, always - get involved in your life.Stay involved. It only comes round once.

Weight loss is a never ending struggle for most men over 50. Most of the weight loss products available on the market today just don't work. A few work in the event you stick to a regime which includes physical exercise, eating properly, and taking their diet supplement. Not many products work alone to give you the results you would like to achieve.

So if your struggling with weight loss, here are 7 tips to follow that get results.

Set Yourself Up For Success

Plan on using small manageable steps. Approach your diet changes gradually and with a focused commitment. Keeping your diet focused and manageable allows for a healthy diet.

The Key Is Moderation

Don't think of your diet as an all or nothing deal. The key to healthy dieting is moderation. Don't fall for the fad diet hype, for a healthy body we need a balance of minerals, vitamins, fiber, fat, protein, and carbohydrates.

Eat Whole Grains And Healthy Carbs

For long lasting energy, choose fiber sources and healthy carbohydrates. Whole grains protect our bodies against antioxidants that help to fight off diabetes, certain cancers, and heart disease. Simply put for a healthier heart eat more whole grains.

A Necessary Ingredient To Any Diet - Water

Waste products and toxins are stored in our bodies. Water makes up about seventy five percent of our body and helps to flush our systems. Make sure to drink 7 to 8 glasses of water daily to remove the waste products and toxins in your body.

Limit Your Intake Of Sugar And Salt

In moderation it's okay to enjoy sweets, but lessen your sugar intake. Sugar adds to health problems such as, depression, headaches, diabetes and arthritis. The same goes for salt, when dieting most of us consume to much salt. You needs to limit yourself to one teaspoon of salt daily for all meals.

Exercise

We need to exercise daily to keep active. There are numerous benefits to exercising daily. One of the most important is that with regular exercise you will make healthy food choices a habit.

Avoid Unhealthy Foods

Eliminate or reduce from your diet saturated fats. These fats are primarily found in whole milk dairy products and red meat. In addition, you may want to eliminate or reduce your trans fat intake. Trans fat is found in snack foods, cookies, crackers and among other oils, shortenings and processed foods.

Americans today are living life on the fast track. Most of the internet searches are for fast or easy weight loss. While most of the information is geared towards women, men are also interested and in need of health and fitness tips.

Men have the advantage where they can lose weight much easier than women. There are many different health and fitness programs out there for men. Yoga and Pilates are not just for women anymore. There are exercise videos that focus on Yoga and Pilates for Men. There are different types of home exercise equipment that are low cost and easy to use. You just need to have the motivation to follow through with your plans for a healthier life.

Heart Disease, Diabetes, prostate cancer, and other health issues are a rising concern for men. These reasons can and should be a good source of motivation for men today. Men can follow these health and fitness tips to lose weight and get healthy and fit.

Starting out the day with a healthy breakfast helps to kick start metabolism and keeps blood sugar levels even. It also gives a person more energy. When, a man, eats breakfast, he is less likely to eat larger portions of unhealthy food later in the day. Eating plenty of fiber rich foods is important to fill up and feel satisfied between meals. Try to eat whole grains - whole wheat bread, potatoes, and brown rice, instead of white bread, white rice, and pasta - that are simple starches and turn right into sugar. The whole grains take longer to digest and can assist with maintaining lean muscle tissue.

Men are able to eat larger portions of protein than women. They should still concentrate on eating lean proteins such as chicken, turkey, and fish on a daily basis instead of red meat. They should also make sure to eat plenty of fruits and vegetables.

Men can also benefit from portion control and watching their portion sizes. Eating smaller meals more frequently throughout the day as opposed to eating the three traditional square meals a day really does help to keep the metabolism running smoothly and helps to build lean muscle tissue.

The best way to lose weight is with a combination of cardio, strength training and a healthy diet. But, the cornerstone of most weight loss programs is cardio. Exercising on a daily basis is a good way to get in shape and boost metabolism. Many men are concerned about building muscle and may only concentrate on strength training. Cardio is necessary in any fitness program because:

1) It helps you burn more calories in a one sitting. Getting your heart rate up means your blood is pumping, you're breathing hard, you're sweating and burning calories.

2) With many cardio exercises, you can burn 100 to 500 calories depending on how hard you work, how long you exercise and how much you weigh.

3) Burning calories with exercise means you don't have to cut as many calories from your diet.

4) You can do cardio exercise most days of the week without worrying about injury or over training.

Nutritional supplements can be used in conjunction with eating healthy foods and exercise to build lean muscle. There are many supplements out there designed especially for men and their uni☐ue health and fitness needs. They are not meant to be a shortcut to weight change, and taking too much of any one supplement can pose serious health risks. The good news is that average person is unlikely to take so much of a nutrient that they run into trouble. But it's always wise to check in with a doctor before you start using a supplement regularly. And that's definitely true if you're using any supplement in high doses or for prolonged periods of time.

Men and women oftentimes have different health and exercise agendas in mind. Take for example the men.

Most men are more concerned about building up their muscles. They want to look bigger (so as not to be cajoled as being feminine or female-like in form) not fatter, definitely.

For men following this rule, it is very important that they forget this myth of a mantra, "No pain, no gain." Muscle build-up does not come overnight. Discipline is the key to achieving the muscular, well-toned look. Yet discipline does not mean making the body suffer painfully and and adding extra stress from ill-advised exercise.

In any physical activity, the body needs to start slow. Warm-ups are probably the most important part in any exercise program.

The men should try out weight-gaining exercises that they enjoy. Once the fitness plan is put into action by both the body and the mind, the men should gradually increase the amount of weights that they use.

Besides the build-up of muscles, the men may want to think about other forms of weight training for the control of body weight and body fat.

Aerobic training activities are also good for the men. Weight training coupled with aerobics makes for a well-balanced fitness program.

Some aerobic forms of exercises include cycling, jogging, Frisbee-throwing, basically sports that work up the cardiovascular system.

Beginners do not need to be overly enthusiastic about any kind of fitness plan. A safe fitness plan is one that is practiced gradually until the body conforms to the schedule.

As I said earlier, discipline is the key. Overexertion will only make your body lose in the end to stress and injuries.

Before going into any exercise plan, it is highly recommended that the men consult their doctors first. Remember, overall health is not just exercise. Proper nutrition plays an important factor as well.

Thank you

Thank you so much to each of my readers for investing your time to read this book!

If you liked the book, please take a few minutes to post an review

© 2018 by Annika Reinert Allrights reserved

All rights Reserved no part of this publication or the information in it may bequoted from or reproduced in any form by means such otherwise without prior written permission of the copy right holder.

Disclaimer

Although the author and publisher have made every effort to ensure that the information in this book was correct at press time, the author and publisher do not assume and hereby disclaim any liability to any party for any loss, damage, or disruption caused by errors or omissions, whether such errors or omissions result from negligence, accident, or any other cause.

Impressum/Publisher

Julian Schomburg

Dünnwalder Grenzweg 4

DE-51375 Leverkusen

Coverfoto: Depositphotos

Made in the USA
Coppell, TX
18 November 2020